AVOIDING AUTISM

(AUTISM SPECTRUM DISORDER)

How avoiding exposure to blue light at night may reduce the risk for having an autistic child

Richard L. Hansler PhD

ISBN-10:1718946090
ISBN-13:9781718946095

Acknowledgments

I want to thank my wife, Wanda Hansler, for her willingness to let me pursue my book-writing venture at an age when most men are retired. I also want to thank my children and grandchildren for their support and love. I also wish to acknowledge the support of my partners in Photonic Developments LLC, Dr. Edward Carome, Vilnis Kubulins, Dr. Martin Alpert, and Daniel Carome. I also owe a debt of gratitude for my daughter, Susan Thomsen, who edited the manuscript and Mark Thomsen, her husband, who designed the cover.

Forward

There is evidence that the chance of having an autistic child depends on both the parents' genes and on environmental factors. The goal of this book is to examine what environmental factors can be controlled to minimize the risk. One factor that has not been discussed until very recently is the impact of light, especially blue light, on a pregnant woman. If her eyes are exposed to blue light in the hours before bedtime, it prevents her body from producing melatonin. Since melatonin protects the brain of the developing fetus, this lack of melatonin may increase the risk for brain damage that may in turn contribute to the development of autism. We will be looking at the science behind this new idea. We will also look at how simple changes in lifestyle can minimize this risk.

Our motive here is to reduce the risk for Autism Spectrum Disorder (ASD). It should be said, however, that having a child with ASD can be a source of great joy. The attitude of the parents becomes all important. I guess all parents hope their child will develop "normally". When that doesn't happen, accepting reality and rejoicing in every achievement rather than grieving over losses, can make a huge difference. If you ask the question," Why me?", the answer may come back " Who better?" Raising an ASD child to be everything he or she can be may be an extremely challenging experience. It may also add depth and meaning to your life beyond your expectations.

Table of Contents

Introduction

There is a great deal of evidence that melatonin is good for everyone. This is especially true for both mother and child, especially before and during pregnancy. The mother's melatonin protects her unborn baby from brain damage. Exposing the eyes to light, especially blue light in the hours before bedtime, stops the body from producing melatonin. This lack of melatonin during crucial or critical times during gestation may result in brain damage. Until very recently, this potential cause for autism has been ignored.

The lack of melatonin has been shown to increase the risk for heart disease, diabetes, obesity, Alzheimer's disease and several forms of cancer. In 2005, our small group of physicists at John Carroll University developed light bulbs that do not emit blue light, glasses that block blue light and filters for screens of mobile devices that also block blue light. They are available on our website www.lowbluelights.com. We sell them with a money-back guarantee mostly to people who want to improve their sleep. More than 90 percent of purchasers report an improvement.

My hope is that the use of our products will become pervasive so that their benefits will not only help people to sleep, but also reduce the incidence of

deadly diseases. My hope is that pregnant women will also protect the developing brain of the fetus and potentially reduce the incidence of autism. Human behavior can change (for example hardly anyone smokes anymore, especially during pregnancy). Be the first in your crowd to switch to lowbluelights light bulbs or to wear cool orange glasses in the evening.

CHAPTER 1

What is Autism Spectrum Disorder?

[Note: Rather than foot-noting references, the abstract of the referenced paper may be found at <u>www.pubmed.gov</u>, a government data base. Simply put the number in parenthesis in the pubmed search box]

According to the National Institute of Mental Health

Autism spectrum disorder (ASD) is the name for a group of developmental disorders. ASD includes a wide range, "a spectrum," of symptoms, skills, and levels of disability.

People with ASD often have these characteristics:

- Ongoing social problems that include difficulty communicating and interacting with others
- Repetitive behaviors as well as limited interests or activities
- Symptoms that typically are recognized in the first two years of life

- Symptoms that hurt the individual's ability to function socially, at school or work, or other areas of life

Some people are mildly impaired by their symptoms, while others are severely disabled. Treatments and services can improve a person's symptoms and ability to function. Families with concerns should talk to their pediatrician about what they've observed and the possibility of ASD screening. According to the <u>Centers for Disease Control and Prevention (CDC)</u> around 1 in 68 children has been identified with some form of ASD.

What is the difference between Asperger's syndrome and ASD?

In the past, Asperger's syndrome and Autistic Disorder were separate disorders. They were listed as subcategories within the diagnosis of "Pervasive Developmental Disorders." However, this separation has changed. The latest edition of the manual from the American Psychiatric Association, the *Diagnostic and Statistical Manual of Mental Disorders (DSM-5),* does not highlight subcategories of a larger disorder. The manual includes the range of characteristics and severity within one category. People whose symptoms were previously diagnosed as Asperger's syndrome or Autistic Disorder are now included as part of the category called Autism Spectrum Disorder (ASD).

Signs and Symptoms

Parents or doctors may first identify ASD behaviors in infants and toddlers. School staff may recognize these behaviors in older children. Not all people with ASD will show all of these behaviors, but most will show several. There are two main types of behaviors: "restricted / repetitive behaviors" and "social communication / interaction behaviors."

Restrictive / repetitive behaviors may include:

- Repeating certain behaviors or having unusual behaviors
- Having overly focused interests, such as with moving objects or parts of objects
- Having a lasting, intense interest in certain topics, such as numbers, details, or facts.

Social communication / interaction behaviors may include:

- Getting upset by a slight change in a routine or being placed in a new or overly stimulating setting
- Making little or inconsistent eye contact
- Having a tendency to look at and listen to other people less often

- Rarely sharing enjoyment of objects or activities by pointing or showing things to others
- Responding in an unusual way when others show anger, distress, or affection
- Failing to, or being slow to, respond to someone calling their name or other verbal attempts to gain attention
- Having difficulties with the back and forth of conversations
- Often talking at length about a favorite subject without noticing that others are not interested or without giving others a chance to respond
- Repeating words or phrases that they hear, a behavior called *echolalia*
- Using words that seem odd, out of place, or have a special meaning known only to those familiar with that person's way of communicating
- Having facial expressions, movements, and gestures that do not match what is being said
- Having an unusual tone of voice that may sound sing-song or flat and robot-like
- Having trouble understanding another person's point of view or being unable to predict or understand other people's actions.

People with ASD may have other difficulties, such as being very sensitive to light, noise, clothing, or temperature. They may also experience sleep problems, digestion problems, and irritability.

ASD is unique in that it is common for people with ASD to have many strengths and abilities in addition to challenges.

Strengths and abilities may include:

- Having above-average intelligence – the CDC reports 46% of ASD children have above average intelligence
- Being able to learn things in detail and remember information for long periods of time
- Being strong visual and auditory learners
- Excelling in math, science, music, or art.

Diagnosing ASD

Doctors diagnose ASD by looking at a child's behavior and development. Young children with ASD can usually be reliably diagnosed by age two.

Older children and adolescents should be evaluated for ASD when a parent or teacher raises concerns based on watching the child socialize, communicate, and play.

Diagnosing ASD in adults is not easy. In adults, some ASD symptoms can overlap with symptoms of other mental health disorders, such as schizophrenia or attention deficit hyperactivity disorder (ADHD). However, getting a correct diagnosis of ASD as an adult can help a person understand past difficulties, identify his or her strengths, and obtain the right kind of help.

Diagnosis in young children is often a two-stage process:

Stage 1: General Developmental Screening during Well-Child Checkups

Every child should receive well-child check-ups with a pediatrician or an early childhood health care provider. The Centers for Disease Control and Prevention (CDC) recommends specific ASD screening be done at the 18- and 24-month visits.

Earlier screening might be needed if a child is at high risk for ASD or developmental problems. Those at high risk include children who:

- Have a sister, brother, or other family member with ASD
- Have some ASD behaviors
- Were born premature, or early, and at a low birth weight.

Parents' experiences and concerns are very important in the screening process for young children. Sometimes the doctor will ask parents questions about the child's behaviors and combine this information with his or her observations of the child. Children who show some developmental problems during this screening process will be referred for another stage of evaluation.

Stage 2: Additional Evaluation

This evaluation is with a team of doctors and other health professionals with a wide range of specialties who are experienced in diagnosing ASD. This team may include:

- A developmental pediatrician—a doctor who has special training in child development
- A child psychologist and/or child psychiatrist—a doctor who knows about brain development and behavior
- A speech-language pathologist—a health professional who has special training in communication difficulties.

The evaluation may assess:

- Cognitive level or thinking skills
- Language abilities
- Age-appropriate skills needed to complete daily activities independently, such as eating, dressing, and toileting.

Because ASD is a complex disorder that sometimes occurs along with other illnesses or learning disorders, the comprehensive evaluation may

include:
- Blood tests
- Hearing test

The outcome of the evaluation will result in recommendations to help plan for treatment.

Diagnosis in older children and adolescents

Older children whose ASD symptoms are noticed after starting school are often first recognized and evaluated by the school's special education team. The school's team may refer these children to a health care professional.

Parents may talk with a pediatrician about their child's social difficulties including problems with subtle communication. These subtle communication issues may include understanding tone of voice, facial expressions, or body language. Older children may have trouble understanding figures of speech, humor, or sarcasm. Parents may also find that their child has trouble forming friendships with peers. The pediatrician can refer the child for further evaluation and treatment.

Diagnosis in adults

Adults who notice the signs and symptoms of ASD should talk with a doctor and ask for a referral for an ASD evaluation. While testing for ASD in adults is still being refined, adults can be referred to a psychologist or psychiatrist with ASD expertise. The expert will ask about concerns, such as social interaction and communication challenges, sensory issues, repetitive behaviors, and restricted interests. Information about the adult's developmental history will help in making an accurate diagnosis, so an ASD evaluation may include talking with parents or other family members.

Risk Factors

Scientists don't know the exact causes of ASD, but research suggests that genes and environment play important roles.

Risk factors include:

- Gender—boys are more likely to be diagnosed with ASD than girls
- Having a sibling with ASD
- Having <u>older parents</u> (a mother who was 35 or older, and/or a father who was 40 or older when the baby was born)

- Genetics—about 20% of children with ASD also have certain genetic conditions. Those conditions include Down syndrome, fragile X syndrome, and tuberous sclerosis among others.

In recent years, the number of children identified with ASD has increased. Experts disagree about whether this shows a true increase in ASD since the guidelines for diagnosis have changed in recent years as well. Also, many more parents and doctors now know about the disorder, so parents are more likely to have their children screened, and more doctors are able to properly diagnose ASD, even in adulthood.

End of quote from National Institute of Mental Health

According to The Autism Society

There is no known single cause for autism spectrum disorder, but it is generally accepted that it is caused by abnormalities in brain structure or function. Brain scans show differences in the shape and structure of the brain in children with autism compared to in neurotypical children. Researchers do not know the exact cause of autism but are investigating a number of theories, including the links among heredity, genetics and medical problems.

In many families, there appears to be a pattern of autism or <u>related disabilities</u>, further supporting the theory that the disorder has a genetic basis. While no one gene has been identified as causing autism, researchers are searching for irregular segments of genetic code that children with autism may have inherited. It also appears that some children are born with a susceptibility to autism, but researchers have not yet identified a single "trigger" that causes autism to develop.

Other researchers are investigating the possibility that under certain conditions, a cluster of unstable genes may interfere with brain development, resulting in autism. Still other researchers are investigating problems during pregnancy or delivery as well as environmental factors such as viral infections, metabolic imbalances and exposure to chemicals.

End of material from Autism Society website.

Prevalence of ASD

A January 2, 2018 study found

"Autism prevalence plateaus among children, adolescents"

There was no significant increase in the prevalence of autism spectrum disorder among children and adolescents between 2014 and 2016, according to data recently published in *JAMA*.

"Previous surveys have reported a steady increase in ASD prevalence in U.S. children over the past 2 decades," Guifeng Xu, MD, of the department of epidemiology at the University of Iowa College of Public Health, and colleagues wrote.

Researchers analyzed results from 30,502 National Health Interview Survey participants aged 3 to 17 years and found:

- The weighted prevalence of ASD was 2.41% (95% CI, 2.17-2.65);

- In 2014, the prevalence of ASD was 2.24% (95% CI, 1.89-2.59); in 2015 the prevalence was 2.41% (95% CI, 1.98-2.84); in 2016 prevalence was

2.58% (95% CI, 2.14-3.01) (*P* for trend = .23);

- The prevalence of ASD was 1.22% (95% CI, 0.98-1.47) in girls and 3.54% (95% CI, 3.14-3.95) in boys; and

- The prevalence of ASD was 2.71% (95% CI, 2.36-3.05) in non-Hispanic white children and teenagers; 2.36% (95% CI, 1.66-3.07) in non-Hispanic black children and teenagers; and 1.78% (95% CI, 1.41-2.15) in Hispanic children and teenagers.

"Changes in nonetiologic factors (such as diagnostic criteria, public awareness and referral), as well as in etiologic factors (including genetic and environmental risk factors), have been postulated to account for the previously observed increase in ASD prevalence," Xu and colleagues wrote. "Continued monitoring of the prevalence and investigation of changes in risk factors are warranted."

<u>Regression in ASD</u>

Regression is one of the most difficult-to-accept aspects of autism. In up to 50% of cases, a child will appear to be developing completely normally, making all the landmarks that doctors use to determine normal development, and then suddenly begins to regress. A child will have begun speaking and then stops. Social skills, once learned, now disappear. Cognitive ability also declines. Why this happens is poorly understood. It is easy to understand why parents look for some reason why this has occurred. There are1730 technical abstracts on Pubmed dealing with "regression autism", but none offers a clear cause for this regression.

**One possible factor is the use of acetaminophen (Tylenol) if taken by the mother during pregnancy, or also if taken by the child during infancy. Papers by Schultz (20628445) support this idea. Consult your doctor for safer alternatives to acetaminophen for treating fever. [To check this reference go to <u>www.pubmed.gov</u> and put the number in parenthesis in the search box.]

Since melatonin is so effective in protecting the brain, avoiding exposing your child to light that suppresses melatonin during the evening and night may be a way of reducing the risk for regression.

Avoiding evening light exposure should also improve sleep. Much more about maximizing melatonin, later.

Physical changes associated with ASD

1. BRAIN VOLUME RESEARCH

Magnetic resonance imaging and head circumference study of brain size in autism: birth through age 2 years (2005) (16330725)

> Significant enlargement was detected in cerebral cortical volumes but not cerebellar volumes in individuals with autism. Enlargement was present in both white and gray matter, and it was generalized throughout the cerebral cortex. Head circumference (HC) appears normal at birth, with a significantly increased rate of HC growth appearing to begin around 12 months of age.

Brain volume findings in 6-month-old infants at high familial risk for autism (2012) (22684595)

> The authors did not observe significant group differences for head circumference, brain

volume, or abnormalities in radiologic findings from a group of 6-month-old infants at high risk for autism. The authors are unable to conclude that these abnormalities are not present in infants who later go on to receive a diagnosis of autism; rather, abnormalities were not detected in a large group at high familial risk. Future longitudinal studies of the infant brain imaging study group will examine whether brain volume differs in infants who go on to develop autism.

Early brain development in infants at high risk for autism spectrum disorder (2017) (28202961)

In this prospective neuroimaging study of 106 infants at high familial risk of ASD and 42 low-risk infants, we show that hyperexpansion of the cortical surface area between 6 and 12 months of age precedes brain volume overgrowth observed between 12 and 24 months in 15 high-risk infants who were diagnosed with autism at 24 months. Brain volume overgrowth was linked to the emergence and severity of autistic social deficits. A deep-learning algorithm that primarily uses surface area information from magnetic resonance imaging of the brain of 6-12-month-old individuals predicted the diagnosis of autism in individual high-risk children at 24 months (with a positive predictive value of 81% and a sensitivity of 88%). These findings demonstrate that early brain changes occur during the period in which autistic behaviours are first emerging.

2. REDUCTION OF MELATONIN

A number of recent studies suggest that the increased incidence of ASD may in part be related to mothers' increasing exposure to light, especially blue light, in the evening and during the night. This exposure causes a measurable reduction in the mother's production of melatonin. Melatonin is known to be very beneficial to the developing brain. Maternal melatonin crosses the placental barrier and provides important protection to the developing baby's brain.

It is suggested that neurological damage occurring due to a lack of melatonin may be a factor in the development of ASD. We will be examining the evidence for this and some simple changes in lifestyle that can help to avoid this problem.

CHAPTER 2

The Internal or Circadian Clock

Understanding the Circadian Clock

In order to understand how light affects pregnant women, we need to learn about the internal or circadian clock. According to pubmed.org more than 13,000 technical papers have been published about circadian clocks.

Almost all living things have some means for keeping track of time, which allows them to predict and prepare for the future. It's fun to think of all the ways nature has programmed living organisms to work on a schedule, including seasonal as well as daily schedules.

Perhaps the most striking are the many animals that change their colors. Mammals may change the color of their fur: brown in summer, white in winter. Birds often develop brilliant colors or build nests to attract a mate at the right time of year. Many animals become fertile in the fall or winter, so the young are born in the spring, when the chance of survival is highest. Many birds, animals and even butterflies migrate with the changing seasons. All these activities must be done at the right time.

On a shorter time-scale, the organs in living organisms adjust their activities throughout the 24-hour day. The term "circadian" means literally "about a day". For example, the liver needs to produce bile in connection with when food is consumed. A corned beef sandwich eaten at 11PM may not go down as well as one eaten at noon. The kidneys slow down production of urine at night, which prevents us from waking up every couple of hours. The organs and individual cells throughout the body all have local clocks.

The local clocks are synchronized by the master clock that is located in the hypothalamus at the base of the brain, in what is called the suprachiasmatic nucleus (SCN). The master clock follows a cyclical 24 hour schedule as follows: The master clock is synchronized with the rotation of the earth and is reset every morning when the eyes are exposed to natural daylight, especially blue light. Approximately 12 hours later (in the early evening), the clock sends a signal to the pineal gland to start producing melatonin. This informs melatonin receptors, located in organs and tissues, that it is nighttime, time to rest and renew. The concentration of melatonin in the blood stream gradually increases to a maximum about six hours later, during sleep, and then drops to near zero, about wake up time.

This circadian cycle then repeats itself.

When humans first evolved, we lived near the equator where there are 12 hours of light and 12 hours of darkness year-round. The resetting of the clock occurred when the sun came up. When darkness came, melatonin began flowing. This all worked well until people moved away from the equator. Now the clock also needed to be a calendar and predict the changing seasons.

About a century ago, experiments were done in which people moved into caves or other places where there were no means for telling what time it was. Their so-called "free running" clocks continued to keep them on a daily pattern but with days slightly longer than 24 hours, about 24.4 hours. This is referred to as "Non 24". Blind people experience this same situation. They do not experience the daily resetting of their clock because their eyes are not exposed to light in the early morning. This means they may have melatonin present during the day when they want to be awake, and experience poor sleep at night. It was discovered in the 1990s that taking a small amount of melatonin at the same time every day would keep the internal clock synchronized with the earth's rotation. Vanda, a pharmaceutical company, has developed and patented a drug very similar to melatonin that also will reset the internal clock if taken at the same time every day. Interestingly, they advertise their product by showing its benefits for a blind person.

Genes controlling the master clock

Throughout nature there are internal clocks of many different degrees of sophistication. They are put together in modular fashion, where different modules are added to improve function when adjusting to different circumstances, such as changing light duration when moving away from the equator. The change in the duration of darkness becomes the calendar.

The things that are doing the equivalent of "ticking" in a mechanical clock are genes and proteins produced from the genes. A portion of the DNA strand that is in each cell in the body carries out this time tracking duty. In the simplest clock, a portion of the DNA is "opened" for copying by a promoter gene called "Clock". It is copied by genes called "Per" and "Cry", and a protein is produced which is then gradually eliminated in a chemical process. Each of these steps requires a certain length of time. The master clock is restarted when light exposure of the eyes in the morning sends a signal to the SCN that activates a gene called Rev-erb to restart the process. In humans, the clock is much more complex, involving about 14 genes.

How the circadian clock affects pregnant women

For the pregnant woman, and actually for all of us, it is important to have darkness in the evening and to get early morning exposure to light at about the same time every morning.

The circadian clock is reset by exposure to light. There are special sensors in the retina of the eye called intrinsically photosensitive retinal ganglion cells, written ipRGC. They are different from the rods and cones that provide vision and were not discovered until 2001. Their function is two-fold. They connect to the SCN that incorporates the master clock and to several parts of the brain that control alertness and the size of the iris of the eye. They do not contribute to vision. They respond most strongly to blue light with a peak at about 470 nanometers. It is the exposure of these sensors to the blue component in white light that resets the circadian clock.

To maintain a stable circadian rhythm, it is important to have this daily exposure to light. Daylight is probably the best source, but a brightly lit bathroom or kitchen is also effective. Special light boxes are available as well as "sunrise" lights that come on gradually to wake you.

As mentioned earlier, we evolved near the equator where there are 12 hours of light and 12 hours of darkness. Our internal clock will send a signal to the pineal gland to start making melatonin about 12 hours after having been reset by morning light. But this will happen only if we are in darkness, or, at least, not exposed to blue light in the evening. Even relatively low levels of light at night will significantly reduce the flow of melatonin and thus, change the setting of the internal clock.

According to a number of scientists, a reduction in levels of melatonin and its consequent disruption to the circadian clock will have damaging effects on the body. For example, the lifetime of fruit flies is reduced if they are exposed to continuous resetting of their internal clocks. For a pregnant woman, exposure to light at night will cause a reduction in melatonin and may have a damaging effect on the brain of her developing baby.

This double whammy of reduced melatonin production and disrupted circadian clock (continuous jet lag) is damaging to both sleep and health, including the health of the developing fetus. This is a high price for our 24/7 lifestyle.

We will examine how the exposure of pregnant women to the melatonin-suppressing blue rays from all kinds of light sources, including light bulbs and the glowing screens of electronic devices, may be an up-until-now unidentified factor in the development of autism spectrum disorder.

CHAPTER 3

Genetic Factors

In this chapter, we will examine the evidence that some cases of autism are the result of gene mutations, passed on from one generation to the next.

Introduction

Family genetics study reveals new clues to autism risk

Source: University of Washington Health Sciences/UW Medicine

Largest-ever whole genome autism study yields clues on how autism-linked gene changes arise (2016)

A new study from Autism Speaks' MSSNG program expands understanding of autism's complex causes and may hold clues for the future development of targeted treatments. The report, appearing in *npj Genomic Medicine* is the largest-ever whole genome study of autism, involving 200 children with the condition and both their unaffected parents.

The new research focuses on newly arising, or de novo, gene changes in the germline cells that produce a parent's eggs or sperm. Previous studies have shown that these mutations can be major contributors to autism through their effects on early brain development.

The 600 fully sequenced genomes came from MSSNG (pronounced "missing"), the world's largest collection of autism genomes and a collaborative effort of Autism Speaks and The Hospital for Sick Children (SickKids), in Toronto. More than halfway to its goal of sequencing more than 10,000 autism genomes, MSSNG has made this unprecedented resource freely available for worldwide research into the causes and personalized treatments for autism.

Geneticists Stephen Scherer and Ryan Yuen, of SickKids, led the study team, which also included scientists with the University of Toronto, Google, BGI-Shenzhen (China) and Autism Speaks.

The researchers found:

- An abundance of autism-linked changes in DNA outside of the gene-coding regions of the genome. Traditional genetic testing largely ignores the non-coding regions of the genome -- which make up 98 percent of our DNA. Coding DNA spells out our genes. Non-coding DNA had long been considered "junk," with no known function. Geneticists now appreciate that it helps regulate the activity of our genes. This regulation is particularly crucial for healthy brain development, which involves genes turning on and off at precisely the right times.

"This represents the most comprehensive assessment to date on the contribution of non-coding variants to autism," Dr. Yuen says. "As such, it provides an important road map on how whole genome sequencing can advance autism research in the future."

- A clear difference between the de novo mutations that come from the mother versus the father. The study confirmed previous findings that most autism-linked de novo mutations come from the father and tend to increase with his age.

However, the researchers also found that clustered, or concentrated, stretches of de novo mutations tend to come from the mother.

"This new finding may be evidence that different types of gene-change and gene-repair mechanisms are at work in men versus women," Dr. Yuen says. Indeed, the clustered mutations from the mother tended to occur near stretches of deleted or repeated DNA called copy number variations (CNVs) -- a type of mutation that the research team had previously linked to autism.

In addition to genetic changes in egg and sperm, the analysis turned up autism-associated mutations that likely occurred in the embryo soon after fertilization. "These genetic changes can arise due to environmental insults [such as exposure to toxic chemicals]," Dr. Yuen says.

- A new way to explore epigenetic risk factors for autism. The team also developed new methods to look at changes in the epigenetic control of gene expression. Epigenetics is the study of proteins that wrap around our DNA to help regulate gene activity. These epigenetic controls can be disrupted by some -- perhaps many -- of the environmental influences suspected of increasing autism risk. Examples include exposure to certain pollutants, nutritional deficiencies and inflammation during pregnancy. Using their new test, the researchers found significantly disrupted epigenetic patterns in just over 1 percent of the genomes they analyzed.

- A cascade effect, with one altered gene affecting the expression of many other genes involved in brain development. "Using new statistical methods and the whole genome sequence as a framework, we found genes with mutations that led to a cascade of changes in gene expression," Dr. Yuen says. This may help explain how the hundreds of rare gene changes associated with autism may converge to affect a few vital pathways in early brain development, he notes.

End of material from University of Washington Health Sciences/UW Medicine

Twin Studies

Autism and Sensory Sensitivity

Examining the Association between Autistic Traits and Atypical Sensory Reactivity: A Twin Study (2018)

A new study of more than 12,000 twin pairs suggests that the heritable factors that underlie autism significantly overlap with those that influence unusual sensory responses.

The findings reinforce the idea that <u>sensory sensitivities are a core feature of autism</u>. They also hint that a better understanding of the genetic factors underlying sensory responses could reveal insights into autism.

Still, experts caution that the link is preliminary because the study focused on only one form of sensory sensitivity.

Up to 90 percent of people with autism are either overly sensitive to sound, sight, taste, smell or touch, or barely notice them at all. Some seek out sensations by, for example, spinning in circles or stroking items with particular textures. Since 2013, the "Diagnostic and Statistical Manual of Mental Disorders" has included sensory sensitivities in the list of diagnostic criteria for autism.

The reason for a link between autism and these sensitivities has been unclear. Parents and siblings of people with autism often have milder versions of these features, hinting that the sensitivities may run in families.

"You can't really say whether an association you see is genetic or environmental from a family study, so we thought that [a twin study] could be an informative approach," says Mark Taylor, a postdoctoral fellow in the medical epidemiology and biostatistics department at the Karolinska Institutet in Stockholm, Sweden.

The new work suggests that about 85 percent of the overlap between autism features and sensory sensitivities can be explained by shared genetic factors.

__Family factors:

Taylor and his colleagues analyzed data on autism traits and sensory sensitivities in 3,586 pairs of identical twins and 8,833 pairs of fraternal twins. The data came from the Child and Adolescent Twin Study in Sweden, which follows the development of all twins born in Sweden since 1992.

When the children were 9 or 12 years old, their parents completed a 96-item questionnaire, including 17 items about autism traits and 5 about sensory hypersensitivity. The questions are based on the diagnostic criteria for autism and other conditions.

An analysis of the responses revealed that when one twin in a pair has autism features, the other often has sensory sensitivities; this link is stronger among identical twins than fraternal ones. Because identical twins share all of their genetic material and fraternal twins only about half, the finding suggests that traits related to autism and sensory sensitivity share a genetic basis. The results hold up when the researchers control for the children's sex and age.

By comparing the difference between the scores of identical and fraternal twin pairs, the researchers estimate that genetic factors account for 84 percent of the overlap in traits in girls, and 89 percent in boys.

In the meantime, Taylor and his colleagues are exploring whether sensory sensitivities share genetic factors with other conditions that commonly occur in people with autism, such as anxiety and attention deficit hyperactivity disorder.

Other Twin Studies

Twin studies provide a lot of information about the nature of ASD. Identical twins come from just a single egg and have essentially identical DNA. Fraternal twins come from different eggs and are genetically only slightly more alike than non-twin siblings. The rare occurrence of identical twins in which one has ASD and the other does not, are most interesting to researchers. The fact that in about 90% of the cases of identical twins with ASD, both are affected, supports the belief that ASD is a genetic disorder.

<u>Gene expression research</u>

1. Epigenetics study helps focus search for autism risk factors

January 16, 2018

- By Judith Van Dongen, WSU Spokane Office of Research

SPOKANE, Wash. – Scientists have long tried to

pin down the causes of autism spectrum disorder. Recent studies have expanded the search for genetic links from identifying genes toward epigenetics, the study of factors that control gene expression and looks at chemical modifications of DNA and the proteins associated with it.

The challenge is knowing where to look, given that our genome is comprised of more than three billion nucleotides, or building blocks, of DNA.

Now, a breakthrough study by researchers at Washington State University and elsewhere has brought focus to the search for epigenetic mechanisms related to autism. Published in the Jan. 16 issue of _Science Signaling,_ their work identifies more than 2,000 regulatory regions (DNA regions that control gene expression) involved in learning that are strongly associated with autism. Further study within one of those regions revealed a genetic mutation that is associated with increased risk of developing autism.

"Our proof-of-concept study demonstrates the feasibility of going after genetic components of autism that are outside of genes and may eventually lead to improvements in the diagnosis and treatment of autism," said study co-author Lucia Peixoto, assistant professor of biomedical sciences in the <u>WSU Elson S. Floyd College of Medicine</u>, who conducted the study and analyzed the data.

She said that the majority of human-disease-causing mutations are thought to be outside of genes, which make up only 2 percent of our genome.

Looking beyond genes

An estimated two million Americans are affected by autism. About half of them have learning disabilities, which is why the research team looked toward learning and memory to address their research question. It is known that learning requires epigenetic regulation — changes in the regulatory regions of DNA that lead to changes in gene expression that guide the formation of long-term memories. To identify regulatory regions associated with autism, they hypothesized that the same regulatory regions involved in learning and memory may also be linked to autism.

Researchers conducted a classical conditioning experiment in which mice were placed in a box and given a small shock. Upon being placed in the same box after 24 hours, the mice had learned to associate the box with the unpleasant shock and would freeze. The researchers then analyzed DNA from the hippocampus — a brain area critical to memory — to identify learning-induced changes in chromatin accessibility.

Chromatin helps package the long strands of DNA into a compact, dense shape so it fits inside cells. It opens and closes to allow access to certain genes during transcription, essentially controlling the activity of these genes.

Results from the experiments suggested that learning increases chromatin accessibility at specific places in the genome. To determine the regions where these changes were occurring, the researchers conducted a second experiment using the same design and analyzed the data for gene expression levels. They then developed a new bioinformatics tool called Differential Enrichment Scan. The tool allowed them to look at the combined data sets to pinpoint, with a high degree of confidence, 2,365 regions regulated by learning.

Further analysis using data from the Encyclopedia of DNA Elements consortium confirmed that the regions made accessible during learning are also for the most part accessible during development. Next, the team looked for genes near the identified regions and found that many of them are known risk genes for autism spectrum disorder.

Finally, they tried to find a genetic risk factor for autism within one of the regulatory regions, selecting one that is associated with a well-known autism risk gene, *Shank3*. Within the *Shank3* promoter 6 region they identified a single nucleotide polymorphism (or SNP, a common type of genetic variation) known as rs6010065. Analyzing genomic data from a clinical study of 554 children with autism and 214 healthy controls, they found that rs6010065 is indeed associated with autism spectrum disorder.

"One of the major challenges in the genetics of disease is understanding the role of the vast portions of the genome that regulate gene expression. Our work suggests that studying activity-dependent changes in chromatin accessibility may hold the key to understanding the function of this 'dark matter' of the genome and may provide novel insights into the nature of autism and other neurodevelopmental disorders," said Ted Abel, the Roy J. Carver Chair of Neuroscience and director of the Iowa Neuroscience Institute at the University of Iowa. Abel and Peixoto collaborated on these studies, which were started when both were at the University of Pennsylvania.

Easing the burden

Peixoto said their work opens the door for scientists to delve farther into the other regulatory regions identified in the study, increasing our understanding of the genetic factors involved in autism with learning disability. She said the same approach could also be used to identify regulatory regions that are involved in other behaviors that are disturbed in autism — such as sleep and social interaction — and to look for mutations in those areas.

End of Van Dongen article

2. Lab-grown neurons showcase effects of autism mutations

BY EMILY ANTHES

15 JANUARY 2018

 Neurons derived from people with mutations linked to autism display diverse abnormalities that may help explain the origins of these individuals' features, according to three new studies.

In all three studies, researchers reprogrammed skin cells from individuals with one of these mutations into stem cells that can mature into any cell type. They then turned these induced pluripotent stem (iPS) cells into neurons.

In one study, Lauren Weiss and her colleagues crafted neurons from people who have a mutation in a region of chromosome 16 associated with autism. These neurons display abnormalities in size, shape and function that correspond with features seen in people with the mutations, the team reported[1].

The researchers also reprogrammed skin cells from people with cardiofaciocutaneous syndrome (CFC), a condition often accompanied by intellectual disability and autism. They found problems in the cultures that suggest an imbalance of brain cell types in people with the condition[2].

Another team generated neurons from people with a deletion or duplication of a region of chromosome 15 linked to autism, epilepsy and related conditions. These neurons show abnormalities that could disrupt their signaling, the team found[3].

Together, the studies provide new insight into the cellular consequences of genetic variants associated with autism and related conditions.

Size matters:

Weiss and her colleagues derived neurons from the skin cells of three people with deletions and three with duplications of the 16p11.2 chromosomal region; both types of mutations are associated with autism. The researchers also generated neurons from four typical individuals.

Neurons derived from people with a 16p11.2 deletion have unusually large cell bodies and unusually long dendrites, or signal-receiving branches. By contrast, those from people with a duplication in this region are atypically small and have truncated dendrites.

The results jibe with the observation that people with a 16p11.2 deletion tend to have macrocephaly, or abnormally large heads, whereas those with an extra copy of the region are likely to have microcephaly, or small heads.

Neurons with either type of mutation have fewer synapses, the junctions between neurons, than do those from controls, the researchers found.

The findings help explain certain features in people with a 16p11.2 variant. They also suggest that different genes within the region underlie the disparate features seen in people with a mutation in the region. (The region contains 29 genes.)

"The mechanism for cell size, which we think is likely to be related to macrocephaly and microcephaly, did appear to be distinct from that of synapse density, which seems more likely to be related to behavioral features," says Weiss, associate professor of psychiatry at the University of California, San Francisco.

End of Anthes article

3. Synaptic and transcriptionally downregulated genes are associated with cortical thickness differences in autism (2018) (29483624)

"We conclude that transcriptionally downregulated genes implicated in autism are robustly associated with global changes in cortical thickness variability in children with autism."

Basically this says they are now able to correlate genetic information associated with ASD and measured (by MRI) cortical thickness in different regions of the brain. The cortex is the outer layer of the brain. This is consistent with head circumference variability associated with autism.

<u>Conclusion</u>

As more studies are done regarding the genetic factors affecting autism, the picture is becoming more and more complex. Some conditions can be traced to the presence of just one gene mutation. This is the case with fragile x syndrome and cystic fibrosis. Only about one percent of ASD cases can be attributed to one particular gene mutation or other abnormality. ASD is a range of conditions that appear to arise from a spectrum of genetic factors. In many cases the parental DNA plays a role. Many genetic factors are referred to as *de novo*, or *spontaneous,* where the defect appears in the autistic child but not in either parent. Not only is the genetics complex, environmental factors also play a significant role in ASD.

A person has basically no control over the genetic makeup of their children other than, perhaps, making decisions regarding who to marry and whether to have children. However, one can control exposure to certain environmental factors that a child experiences, both before and after birth.

We want to use our knowledge about specific environmental factors to minimize a child's risk for Autism Spectrum Disorder.

CHAPTER 4

Environmental Factors

This chapter covers a variety of environmental factors that may affect the brain development of the fetus and may be potential contributing factors in the development of Autism Spectrum Disorder.

1. Rubella Vaccination

In recent years, there has been an unfortunate trend against vaccination due to misinformation. In the case of German measles (Rubella), it was thought the disease had been eliminated as of 2004. Sadly, a small number of people refusing vaccination have allowed the disease to survive, endangering the entire population. Rubella is particularly dangerous to preganant women and their developing baby.

From the Centers for Disease Control:

> Rubella is very dangerous for <u>a pregnant woman and her developing baby</u>. Anyone who is not vaccinated against rubella is at risk of getting the disease. Although rubella was declared eliminated from the U.S. in 2004, cases can occur when unvaccinated people are exposed to infected people, mostly through international travel. Women

should make sure they are protected
from rubella before they get pregnant.

Infection with rubella virus causes the
most severe damage when the mother
is infected early in pregnancy, especially
in the first 12 weeks (first trimester).
During 2005-2015, eight babies with
CRS have been reported in the United
States.

Congenital Rubella Syndrome (CRS)

Congenital rubella syndrome (CRS) is a
condition that occurs in a developing
baby in the womb whose mother is
infected with the rubella virus. Pregnant
women who contract rubella are at risk
for miscarriage or stillbirth, and their
developing babies are at risk for severe
birth defects with devastating, lifelong
consequences. CRS can affect almost
everything in the developing baby's
body.

The most common birth defects from
CRS can include:
- Deafness
- Cataracts
- Heart defects
- Intellectual disabilities

- Liver and spleen damage
- Low birth weight
- Skin rash at birth

Less common complications from CRS can include:
- Glaucoma
- Brain damage
- Thyroid and other hormone problems
- Inflammation of the lungs

Although specific symptoms can be treated, there is no cure for CRS. Since there is no cure, it is important for women to get vaccinated before they get pregnant.

Vaccine Recommendations

Women who are planning to become pregnant should check with their doctor to make sure they are vaccinated before they get pregnant.

Because MMR vaccine is an attenuated (weakened) live virus vaccine, pregnant women who are not vaccinated should wait to get MMR vaccine until after they have given birth.

Adult women of childbearing age should avoid getting pregnant for at least four weeks after receiving MMR vaccine.

Pregnant women should NOT get MMR

vaccine.
If you get rubella or are exposed to rubella while you're pregnant, contact your doctor immediately.

End of material from the Center for Disease Control

2. Folic Acid/Multivitamin Supplements

Association of Maternal Use of Folic Acid and Multivitamin Supplements in the Periods Before and During Pregnancy with the Risk of Autism Spectrum Disorder in Offspring (2018) (29299606)

Author's summary:

Of 45□300 children born to 26□702 mothers, 572 (1.3%) received a diagnosis of ASD. Maternal folic acid and/or multivitamin supplement exposure before and during pregnancy <u>reduced the risk of ASD in offspring</u>. Our results are consistent with those from a Norwegian birth cohort study showing that maternal folic acid use from 4 weeks before and 8 weeks into pregnancy is associated with a reduced risk of ASD in offspring This interval is considered relevant to the development of the central nervous system, includes neural tube closure, and is implicated in the development of basic brain structures.

Prenatal vitamins tied to lower autism risk in kids, study finds (HealthDay reporter)

Kids were less likely to be diagnosed with autism if their moms took supplements before pregnancy and while they were expecting, according to a study of just over 45,000 Israeli children.

"Reduced risk of [autism] in offspring is a consideration for public health policy that may be realized by extended use of folic acid and multivitamin supplements during pregnancy," the researchers concluded in the report.

The international team of scientists, led by Stephen Levine from the University of Haifa in Israel, gathered data on tens of thousands of children born in Israel between 2003 and 2007, and followed their progress until 2015.

The team also gathered prescription data, to see whether the kids' mothers had been prescribed folic acid or multivitamin supplements either prior to or during pregnancy.

Women who took supplements prior to pregnancy were 61 percent less likely to have a child diagnosed with autism, compared with moms who didn't take supplements, the researchers found.

In addition, taking supplements during pregnancy was linked to a 73 percent reduced risk of an autism diagnosis, the findings showed.

The overall risk of autism remained low, with only 1.3 percent of the children in the study receiving a diagnosis.

But these study results suggest that taking folic acid and multivitamins could be a way to protect babies against the development of autism, said Tom Frazier, chief science officer for Autism Speaks, a group that promotes advocacy and support for individuals with autism and their families.

Women already are urged to take folic acid during pregnancy to prevent birth defects of the spinal cord and the brain, Frazier said. Multivitamins also are recommended to help cover any nutritional gaps in an expecting mom's diet.

"The study suggests this is not a trivial recommendation. This is something that people really should pay attention to," Frazier said. "The reduction in risk isn't huge, but it isn't small either."

Folic acid plays an essential role in fetal neural development, and a lack of the vitamin could possibly set the stage for later onset of autism, Frazier said. He's not sure how the protective effect of multivitamins might work.

Antiepileptic drugs and folic acid. Contemporary Pediatrics (2018)

A new study suggests that mothers who take medications to control their epileptic seizures without folic acid supplementation during their pregnancy may be placing their unborn children at risk of later displaying autistic traits.

The large-scale Norwegian study was published in *JAMA Neurology* in December 2017. Researchers used the Norwegian Mother and Child Cohort Study to assess the effects of both antiepileptic drugs (AEDs) and folic acid supplementation between June 1999 and December 2008. The women's children were studied at age 18 to 36 months. In the folic acid group, supplementation was given from 4 weeks before to 12 weeks after conception, with plasma folate levels tested at between 17 and 19 weeks' gestation, according to the report. As for the outcomes in children, autistic traits were assessed using the Modified Checklist for Autism in Toddlers and Social Communication Questionnaire.

The research team found that of the 335 children exposed to AEDs in utero, the risk for autistic traits was significantly higher at 18 and 36 months of age when folic acid supplementation was not used in comparison with the mothers who took AEDs and folic acid supplements. In women with untreated epilepsy, 389 children displayed insignificant risks of autistic traits, the report notes. The study suggests that the degree of autistic traits was inversely associated with the plasma folate concentration of the mother during pregnancy, but that the concentration of AEDs was not specifically associated with any degree of autistic traits.

The results suggest that women who take AEDs to treat epilepsy during pregnancy need to mitigate the dangers of these medications with folic acid supplementation even before conception.

Marte Bjørk, MD, of Haukeland University Hospital, Bergen, Norway, led the study and says considering that there are a high number of unplanned pregnancies in women with epilepsy, clinicians should consider advocating for low-dose daily folic acid supplementation in women of childbearing age who take AEDs.

Bjørk says overall prevalence of children exposed to AEDs in utero that later displayed autistic traits was between 26% and 32% when folic acid supplementation was not used. That prevalence dropped to 6% to 9% when folic acid supplementation was used.

At least 0.4 mg daily is generally recommended, with some guidelines going as high as 5 mg for pregnancy. However, Bjørk notes that higher doses of folic acid—5 mg and above—have been associated with other adverse conditions in children.

"I give my female patients on antiepileptic drugs 0.4 mg if there is any chance that they may get pregnant. When they plan pregnancy, I increase the dose to 4 mg and they stay on this dose throughout the first trimester," Bjørk says. "I then lower the dose to 0.4 mg. I also check their blood levels of folate, methylmalonic acid, and B12 regularly."

Bjørk says she hopes the study will emphasize the importance of examining folate levels in women with epilepsy.

3. Overweight and Obesity

High risk for obstructive sleep apnea (OSA) and other sleep disorders among overweight and obese pregnant women (2016) (26330183)

Compared with lean women (<25 kg/m(2)), overweight women (25-29.9 kg/m(2)) had 3.69-fold higher odds of high risk for OSA (95% CI 1.82-7.50). The corresponding aOR for obese women (≥30 kg/m(2)) was 13.23 (95% CI: 6.25-28.01).

Maternal Body Mass Index and Risk of Autism Spectrum Disorders in Offspring: A Meta-analysis (2016) (27687989)

Totally, 6 cohort studies and 1 case-control study involving 8,403 cases and 509,167 participants were included for analysis. The summary RR (95% confidence interval) for ASD in offspring in relation to maternal underweight, overweight, and obesity vs. normal weight during pre-pregnancy or pregnancy, was 1.07 (0.93, 1.23), 1.28 (1.19, 1.36) and 1.36 (1.03, 1.78), respectively. A linear dose-response relationship was found, with a pooled RR of 1.16 (1.01, 1.33) for each $5\,kg/m^2$, increment in maternal BMI. The present study suggests that excessive maternal BMI is associated with increased incidence of ASD.

To paraphrase, "<u>Overweight and obesity increase the probability of having a child with ASD by 28 and 36% respectively</u>".

The previous (OSA) study provides a hint of a mechanism to explain the association. Obstructive sleep apnea reduces the amount of oxygen in the blood when the patient stops breathing, sometimes to dangerous levels. This results in the fetus experiencing a risk for brain damage and possibility for ASD. Melatonin has been shown to be especially beneficial in preventing brain damage caused by hypoxia. This is why it is so important to maximize melatonin by avoiding blue light exposure in the hours before bedtime, especially if the pregnant woman is overweight or obese.

4. Diabetes

What's the autism-diabetes link? Autism
Interactive Network (2006)

Scientists have been trying to tease out the
relationship between a mother's diabetes and
her child's autism in recent years.

Researchers at Kaiser Permanente Southern
California examined the prenatal records of
more than 322,000 mothers; almost 3,400 of
their children were later diagnosed with
autism. In analyzing data, they took into
account other factors that could affect the
results, such as a mother's age, race,
ethnicity, level of education, and history of
heart, lung, kidney or liver disease, or cancer.
They also looked at smoking and weight in a
subset of the mothers. They made those
adjustments to ensure they were only
calculating the effect of diabetes on autism
risk.

They found that moms diagnosed with
gestational diabetes by 26 weeks of
pregnancy were 42 percent more likely to
have a child with autism, compared to women
without diabetes.[1] To put it in perspective, the
risk of having a child with autism is about 1.5
percent; gestational diabetes raises the risk to

a little over 2 percent, according to that study.

Moms' diabetes didn't raise autism risk in some babies

Interestingly, women who were diagnosed with diabetes after 26 weeks of pregnancy did not have a higher risk of having a child with ASD. Perhaps that is because those children were exposed to high blood sugar after a period of critical brain development had passed, or because their mothers' diabetes was mild, the researchers speculated.[1] In the United States, most doctors screen pregnant women for diabetes between their 24th and 28th week of pregnancy because that is when gestational diabetes usually develops.

Also, children whose mothers had Type 2 diabetes did not have a higher autism risk. Those mothers knew they had diabetes before they became pregnant, so they and their doctors could have monitored and controlled their blood sugar during early pregnancy, according to one theory. The lead researcher, biostatistician Anny Hui Xiang, PhD, said, "This is just speculation: perhaps the mom with known diabetes [before pregnancy] can make sure her blood sugar is under control, but the mom who doesn't know she has diabetes will not get treatment until she is diagnosed."

What happens when a mother has obesity *and* diabetes?

Across the country, researchers launched two similar diabetes-autism studies, but with a few crucial differences. One group studied a group of mothers in Boston with a higher rate of obesity and diabetes than average.[2] Being obese raises the risks of developing Type 2 diabetes and gestational diabetes.

"The global epidemics of obesity and diabetes affect all ages, including pregnant women," said Xiaobin Wang, MD, one of the researchers. They wondered: Did having both conditions produce a combined effect that was greater than having just diabetes or obesity alone?

It did. According to this study, mothers who had diabetes and obesity before pregnancy were four times more likely to have a child with autism. Moms who had obesity and gestational diabetes were three times more likely to have a child with ASD. The Boston study was smaller than the one from Kaiser Permanente. Researchers analyzed the pregnancies of 2,734 women; 102 of their babies eventually were diagnosed with autism.

Another study, conducted in Cincinnati, Ohio, reached similar conclusions when examining both obesity and diabetes during pregnancy. This large study involved children seen by developmental pediatricians at Cincinnati Children's Hospital, as well as thousands of children without developmental conditions born in the same region. Expectant mothers who were obese or who had gestational diabetes were 1.5 times more likely to have a child with autism than other mothers in the study. Having both diabetes and obesity doubled the risk of autism in babies.

End of quote from Autism Interactive Network

5. Male Hormones

New Study investigates the molecular basis for male predisposition to autism (2018) <u>Elsevier</u>

Exposure to androgens (male hormones) during brain development alters genes related to autism spectrum disorder (ASD), according to a new study published in *Biological*

Psychiatry. Using male human cells, researchers at the University of Strasbourg, France, identified key genes that are regulated by testosterone and that contribute to the risk for autism, generating important insight into how male hormones might contribute to the increased male susceptibility to ASD.

The findings provide a clue as to why ASD affects boys about four times as much as girls. Male fetuses produce androgens during critical stages of brain development when cells divide and develop into neurons. The researchers showed that androgens increase the spread of cells and prevent them from death, which could predispose boys to ASD by contributing to the excessive brain growth that occurs in people with ASD during the first years of life.

"Understanding the mechanisms for the male preponderance for autism is like pulling on a loose thread. It could help to 'unravel' important mechanisms contributing to autism risk," said John Krystal, Editor of Biological Psychiatry. Identifying a role of androgens in this risk could be important for prevention or the development of potential treatments for ASD.

In the study, co-senior authors Jean-Louis Mandel, M.D., Ph.D., and Amélie Piton, Ph.D., and colleagues used human pluripotent neural stems cells to model the cells that generate neurons during <u>brain development</u>. Treatment with the testosterone metabolite DHT led to subtle changes in the expression of about 200 genes, several of which have previously been associated with ASD. Some of the genes that were most affected by DHT treatment included NRCAM, which has been linked to the brain abnormalities and symptoms in ASD, and FAM107A, which is increased in people with ASD. FAM107A also appeared to play a part in androgen's ability to increase cell numbers in the study.

"These effects of male hormones may therefore contribute to the increased sensitivity of the male brain to develop ASD when also exposed to other genetic or environmental factors," said Dr. Piton, suggesting that the biological explanation for the sex-specific inequality of ASD points to a predisposition in males, rather than a protective effect in females.

In addition to providing a clue into the male susceptibility to ASD, Dr. Piton says that the list of genes that were altered by androgens in the study might be useful to identify new genes that might be involved in ASD or in other diseases that occur more often in males.

6. Alcohol

Any drinking during pregnancy increases the odds of fetal alcohol syndrome, but the risk to the fetus is highest if a pregnant woman drinks during the second half of her first trimester of pregnancy, a new study finds.

For every one drink per day increase in alcohol intake during that crucial period, a woman's baby was 25 percent more likely to have an abnormally shaped lip, 12 percent more likely to have a smaller-than-normal head and 16 percent more likely to have low birth weight — all early signs of fetal alcohol syndrome, the study showed.

"The take-home message is that there's not a low threshold level below which drinking alcohol doesn't raise the risk," of fetal alcohol syndrome, said study author Dr. Christina Chambers of the University of California, San Diego. "This supports the surgeon general's recommendation that drinking be avoided entirely."

In 2004, the Surgeon General of the United States issued this warning:

> Alcohol consumed during pregnancy increases the risk of alcohol related birth defects, including growth deficiencies, facial abnormalities, central nervous system impairment, behavioral disorders, and impaired intellectual development. No amount of alcohol consumption can be considered safe during pregnancy

Autism and attention-deficit/hyperactivity disorder among individuals with a family history of alcohol use disorders (2014) (25139954)

Recent studies suggest de novo mutations may involve the pathogenesis of autism and attention-deficit/hyperactivity disorder (ADHD). Based on the evidence that excessive alcohol consumption may be associated with an increased rate of de novo mutations in germ cells (sperms or eggs), we examine here whether the risks of autism and ADHD are increased among individuals with a family history of alcohol use disorders (AUDs). The standardized incidence ratios (SIRs) of autism and ADHD among individuals with a biological parental history of AUDs were 1.39 (95% CI 1.34-1.44) and 2.19 (95% CI 2.15-2.23), respectively, compared to individuals without an affected parent. Among offspring whose parents were diagnosed with AUDs before their birth, the corresponding risks were 1.46 (95% CI 1.36-1.58) and 2.70 (95% CI 2.59-2.81), respectively. Our study calls for extra surveillance for children with a family history of AUDs, and further studies examining the underlying mechanisms are needed.

[A standardized incidence ratio of 1.39 means the number of affected births will be 39% higher for AUD parents than for non AUD parents.]

7. Smoking

A 2015 analysis (25432101) of multiple studies concluded there <u>is no evidence that parent's smoking increases the risk of autism.</u>

However, the following article suggests potential links between maternal smoking and the development of mental health problems (including ADHD) in the child. **From Healthyday.com website** (2010) HealthDay News

A woman who smokes while pregnant increases her baby's risk of developing psychiatric problems in childhood and young adulthood, a new Finnish study suggests.

While there's plenty of evidence that smoking during pregnancy puts unborn children at risk for long-term health problems such as asthma, ear infections and respiratory disease, this research is among the first to find a connection between prenatal smoking and an increased risk for mental illnesses, such as attention-deficit/hyperactivity disorder (ADHD) and depression, in the mother's offspring.

Researchers at Turku University Hospital in Finland analyzed the birth records of more than 175,000 Finnish children born in the late 1980s, as well as their use of psychotropic medications as children and young adults.

Children exposed to prenatal smoking were 32 percent more likely overall to have taken a psychiatric drug than children whose mothers didn't smoke during pregnancy, the researchers found. The risk was even higher in the offspring of women who smoked more than a pack a day while pregnant. Their kids were 44 percent more likely to use psychiatric drugs than children whose moms didn't smoke.

Study author Mikael Ekblad said animal studies have shown that prenatal nicotine exposure interferes with the development of fetal brain cells. "In our previous study, published in the *Journal of Pediatrics* in February 2010, we found that prematurely born infants exposed to prenatal smoking had smaller frontal and cerebellar brain volumes than the unexposed infants. These brain regions are important for normal cognitive development," said Ekblad, a medical student and pediatric researcher.

The researchers collected data on all children born in Finland from 1987 through 1989. In addition to information about maternal smoking, they looked at gestational age, birth weight and five-minute Apgar scores. Using records from Finland's Social Insurance Institution, they also examined the children's use of psychotropic medications between 1994 and 2007.

Roughly 12 percent of the young adults had used psychiatric medications, and of this group, about 19 percent had mothers who smoked during their pregnancies.

The researchers found that exposure to prenatal smoking increased the risk for using all psychotropic drugs, but especially ADHD medications, antidepressants and drugs to treat addiction. For example, kids whose mothers smoked more than a pack of cigarettes a day were two and a half times more likely to take stimulants for ADHD than kids whose moms didn't smoke during pregnancy.

The risk for all medication use was similar in males and females, and remained after adjusting for risk factors at birth, such as Apgar scores and birth weight.

Since mental illness often runs in families, the researchers also controlled for a possible genetic connection by analyzing records of the mother's psychiatric inpatient care prior to giving birth. "One of the strengths of our study is that we could control for maternal mental health diseases," said Ekblad, who added that the genetic effect is higher in psychiatric problems that require hospitalization.

"This is an interesting study which raises the important possibility that prenatal exposure to smoking may pose additional risks that have not been identified to date, but based on the information available so far, the effect seems to be small," said Neil Grunberg, a professor of medical psychology, clinical psychology and neuroscience at the Uniformed Services University of the Health Sciences in Bethesda, Md.

Grunberg also questioned whether the study adequately controlled for possible genetic and environmental factors. "In the U.S., there is a high correlation between smoking and psychological disorders," said Grunberg. In addition, many people have a family history of psychiatric disorders, even though they themselves have never been diagnosed with one, he said.

8. Tylenol/Acetaminophen

From "Working Mother" website:

Although generally considered safer than taking ibuprofen or aspirin, the scientific community, in recent years, has come to find that acetaminophen (Tylenol) use during pregnancy may pose its own set of health risks to the child. Now, a new peer-reviewed article is claiming that the use of the drug, also known as paracetamol, is linked to Attention

Deficit Hyperactivity Disorder (ADHD), Autism Spectrum Disorder (ASD) and lower IQ.

To write the review, which is published in the journal *Hormones and Behavior,* researchers examined 64 recent studies, and found nine that suggested an association between acetaminophen use while pregnant and babies' brain development

The review also found that the longer acetaminophen is taken by an expectant mother, the higher her child's risk of developing ADHD, ASD or a lower IQ. The link between taking acetaminophen and negative neurological outcomes for the child was the strongest for hyperactivity and attention-related effects.

A wonderful organization associated with Harvard Medical School and the Massachusetts General Hospital is the **Center for Women's Mental Health.** They are especially concerned about the impact of the environment on childbirth and maintain information in a drug registry. If in doubt about the drug you are taking while pregnant, contact them.

9. Exposure to Mobile Phone Radiation

Mobile phone radiation induces mode-dependent DNA damage in a mouse spermatocyte-derived cell line: a protective role of melatonin. (2015) (23995262)

https://www.ncbi.nlm.nih.gov/pubmed/23952262

Abstract

PURPOSE:

To evaluate whether exposure to mobile phone radiation (MPR) can induce DNA damage in male germ cells.

MATERIALS AND METHODS:

A mouse spermatocyte-derived GC-2 cell line was exposed to a commercial mobile phone handset once every 20 min in standby, listen, dialed or dialing modes for 24 h. DNA damage was determined using an alkaline comet assay.

RESULTS:

The levels of DNA damage were significantly increased following exposure to MPR in the listen, dialed and dialing modes. Moreover, there were significantly higher increases in the dialed and dialing modes than in the listen mode. Interestingly, these results were consistent with the radiation intensities of these modes. However, the DNA damage effects of MPR in the dialing mode were efficiently attenuated by melatonin pretreatment.

CONCLUSIONS:

These results regarding mode-dependent DNA damage have important implications for the safety of inappropriate mobile phone use by males of reproductive age and also suggest a simple preventive measure: Keeping mobile phones as far away from our body as possible, not only during conversations but during 'dialed' and 'dialing' operation modes. Since the 'dialed' mode is actually part of the standby mode, mobile phones should be kept at a safe distance from our body even during standby operation. Furthermore, the protective role of melatonin suggests that it may be a promising pharmacological candidate for preventing mobile phone use-related reproductive impairments.

10. Early Changes in Lifestyle – Start before you are pregnant!!!

Neurodevelopmental Hypothesis about the Etiology of Autism Spectrum Disorders (2017) (28744208)

Etiology means origin. This article reviews the evidence that damage to the developing brain of the fetus occurs about the time the woman notices her period is late and she may be pregnant. This is why it is so important that the changes in lifestyle to reduce risk for ASD (that we will discuss in Chapter 6) are made at the time you decide to try to become pregnant. Waiting until you know you are pregnant may have already increased your risk for having a child with ASD.

11. Exposure to artificial light at night

A more recently identified factor in the development of a child with ASD is the exposure of the parents to blue light in the evening. The blue component of artificial light is known to cause a reduction in melatonin production. Prior to conception, melatonin is known to have beneficial effects in creating a healthy egg and sperm. During pregnancy, the fetus relies entirely on the mother's melatonin. Thus, any reduction in maternal melatonin (as is caused by exposure to artificial light in the evening) may be potentially damaging to the baby's developing brain.

By avoiding blue light at night, the parents can reduce the risk of having a child with ASD.

In the next chapter, we will examine in greater detail the important role of melatonin both prior to and during fetal development.

CHAPTER 5

Melatonin and the Child's Developing Brain

Introduction

A milestone 2017 paper (29346266) from Korea, **"The relationship between autism spectrum disorder and melatonin during fetal development"**, describes how the development of the child's brain is protected by the mother's melatonin. Melatonin crosses the placental barrier and enters the fetal circulation. The fetus does not begin to make melatonin until around birth. This means the baby's developing brain depends almost entirely on the melatonin concentration in the mother's blood.

An additional paper (2016) from the Netherlands by Braam et al, provides experimental support (for the first time) for the concept that lack of melatonin in the parents increases the risk for ASD in their offspring. The paper may be found at:

https://www.biorxiv.org/content/biorxiv/early/2016/04/02/046722.full.pdf

In this study, the amount of melatonin metabolite found in overnight urine was measured for mothers of ASD children compared to mothers of children without ASD. The ASD mothers produced only about 2/3 the amount of melatonin as the non-ASD mothers.

This study provides confirmation that maximizing natural melatonin will reduce the incidence of ASD.

It is well understood that exposure to blue light in the evening suppresses natural melatonin production. While there is not yet a proven causative relationship between exposure to blue light and an increased incidence of ASD, an association between them appears to be evident. A variety of artificial light sources, including LED lit screens on computers, smart phones and ordinary light bulbs, are rich in blue rays. The rise in the incidence of ASD parallels the rise in the use of household devices with LED bulbs and of electronic devices with LED lighted screens.

In other words, a pregnant woman's exposure to artificial light at night causes reduced melatonin production and thus, increases the chance of developing Autism Spectrum Disorder in her baby.

Fetal Brain Development (From Whattoexpect.com)

The fetal nervous system — i.e., your baby-to-be's brain and spinal cord — is one of the very first systems to develop. In fact, it's making big strides before you even know you're pregnant.

The parts of your baby's brain

Before we get into the science of fetal brain development, here's a quick anatomy primer on your baby's brain. There are five parts, each responsible for different functions:

1. **Cerebrum:** This is the biggest part of the brain, and it's responsible for thinking, remembering and feeling. This is where the cerebral cortex and its various lobes (including the frontal and temporal lobes) reside.

2. **Cerebellum:** The area in charge of motor control.

3. **Brain stem:** The engine driving many of your baby's most vital functions, including heart rate, breathing and blood pressure.

4. **Pituitary gland:** This pea-sized gland releases hormones into your body that are responsible for growth, metabolism and more.

5. **Hypothalamus:** This area deals with body temperature, hunger and thirst, sleep and emotions.

With the biology lesson out of the way, read on to find out how and when these various parts start developing.

First trimester: Baby starts moving

A mere 16 days after conception, your fetus's neural plate forms (think of it as the foundation of your baby's brain and spinal cord). It grows longer and folds onto itself, until that fold morphs into a groove, and that groove turns into a tube — the neural tube. Once the neural tube closes, at around <u>week 6</u> or <u>week 7</u> of pregnancy, it curves and bulges into three sections, commonly known as the forebrain, midbrain and hindbrain. Just to the rear of the hindbrain sits the part that will soon turn into your baby's spinal cord. Soon, these areas bubble into those five different regions of the brain that we're most familiar with: the cerebrum, cerebellum, brain stem, pituitary gland and the hypothalamus. Of course, all of these fetal brain areas need more time to be fully up and running!

At the same time, special neural cells form and migrate throughout the embryo to form the very beginnings of nerves. Your baby's nervous system is made up of millions upon millions of neurons; each of these microscopic cells have itty-bitty branches coming off of them so that they can connect and communicate with each other. With this comes baby's first synapses, which essentially means baby's neurons can communicate and create early fetal movements...like curling into (you guessed it!) the fetal position.

Other movements follow quickly, with your fetus wiggling his developing limbs at around 8 weeks. By the end of the first trimester, your baby-to-be has garnered quite a repertoire of motion, though you won't be able to feel any of it quite yet. And at about the same time as baby first wiggles his limbs, he begins to develop the sense of touch.

Second trimester: Baby sucks, swallows, blinks and dreams

During the second trimester, steady contractions of baby's diaphragm and chest muscles occur (think of them as practice breathing movements). Baby's first sucking and swallowing impulses kick in around 16 weeks. By 21 weeks, your baby's natural reflexes will allow him to swallow several ounces of amniotic fluid every day. And all of that swallowing means baby's tasting, too – another sense that's now in full gear.

At around 18 weeks of pregnancy, you'll feel baby's first kick (but don't worry if it takes a few weeks longer — that's common, especially among first-time moms). Around the same time, your baby's nerves become covered with myelin, a protective insulation that speeds messages between nerve cells (myelin continues to grow until your baby's first birthday). And at 24 weeks, another big reflex occurs: Blinking.

At the tail-end of trimester two, your little one's brainstem (heart rate, breathing, blood pressure) is almost entirely mature, resting just above the spinal cord but below the cerebral cortex (the last area to mature). By now, the fetal nervous system is developed enough so your baby is startled by loud noises outside the womb — and may even turn his head toward the sound of your voice! Another exciting development: At 28 weeks, fetal brainwave activity features sleep cycles, including REM (the stage when dreaming occurs).

Third trimester: Baby's brain grows

The third trimester is brimming with rapid development of neurons and wiring. Baby's brain roughly triples in weight during the last 13 weeks of gestation, growing from about 3.5 ounces at the end the second trimester to almost 10.6 ounces at term. And it's starting to look different, too: Its formerly once smooth surface is becoming increasingly grooved and indented (like the images of brains you're used to seeing).

At the same time, the cerebellum (motor control) is developing fast — faster now than any other area of the fetal brain (its surface area increases 30-fold in the last 16 weeks of pregnancy!).

All of this growth is big news for the cerebral cortex (thinking, remembering, feeling). Though this important area of the brain is developing rapidly during pregnancy, it really only starts to function around the time a full-term baby is born — and it steadily and gradually matures in the first few years of life, thanks to baby's enriching environment.

Eating to support baby's brain development

Because your baby's nervous system starts developing right out of the starting gates, it's important to consume 400 micrograms of folate (aka folic acid or vitamin B) daily as soon as you think you might want to get pregnant. This nutrient is imperative for fetal cell growth, tissue development and DNA — and consuming enough before (and early in) pregnancy reduces a baby's chance of serious neural tube defects (like spina bifida) by 70 percent. Emerging research in the Journal of the American Medical Association also suggests that the nutrient can <u>reduce the chances your child will be born with an autism spectrum disorder</u> by up to 40 percent. So take your <u>prenatal vitamin</u> (which should have at least 400 mcg), and make sure to eat plenty of <u>folate-rich foods</u> (like leafy greens and whole grains).

Another important nutrient for brain (and eye) development: omega-3 fatty acids, specifically DHA (aka docosahexaenoic acid). Getting enough — especially during your third trimester, when baby's brain is developing the fastest — is vital, since it's a major structural fat in the brain and eyes. The good news:

<u>DHA is found</u> in lots of safe-to-eat fatty, cold water fish (like salmon, trout and cod), along with seaweed and DHA-fortified eggs.

Concern over common household chemicals

Chemicals in everyday personal care and other products found around the house may endanger fetal and child brain development, according to a <u>2016 report in the journal Environmental Health Perspectives</u>. Those of most concern include phthalates, which are found in many beauty products, toiletries and plastics; lead; mercury; certain pesticides used on produce and in home gardens; air pollutants and flame retardants. The important thing is, though, not to worry too much. Talk to your doctor to see if there's anything you can do to reduce baby's risk, but chances are these chemicals won't be an issue and everything will turn out just fine.

End of material from "WhattoExpect.com"

Scientific Evidence of Melatonin's Beneficial Effects

1. Benefits to the egg and sperm

A paper (18339123) from 2004 is titled "**Oxidative stress impairs oocyte quality and melatonin protects oocytes from free radical damage and improves fertilization rate.**" It describes how giving women daily 3mg melatonin by mouth improved in vitro fertilization results.

A paper (18804205) from 2009 is titled "**Melatonin and the ovary: physiological and pathophysiological implications.**" The abstract summarizes the results of this review.as follows:

> Melatonin plays an essential role in the pathogenesis of many reproductive processes. Human pre-ovulatory follicular fluid contains higher concentrations of melatonin than does plasma, and melatonin receptors are present in ovarian granulosa cells. Melatonin has been shown to have direct effects on ovarian function. Reactive oxygen species and apoptosis (cell death) are involved in a number of reproductive events including folliculogenesis (development of the follicule), follicular atresia (degeneration\),

ovulation, oocyte maturation, and corpus luteum (temporary endocrine structure in female ovaries) formation. Melatonin and its metabolites are powerful antioxidants; the primitive and primary function of melatonin may be its actions as a receptor-independent free radical scavenger and a broad-spectrum antioxidant. A large amount of scientific evidence supports a local role of melatonin in the human reproductive processes.

A 2014 study (24628045) is titled "**Oral melatonin supplementation improves oocyte and embryo quality in women undergoing in vitro fertilization-embryo transfer.**"

Abstract

The aim of this study was to evaluate the efficacy of oral melatonin supplementation on oocyte and embryo quality in patients in an assisted reproductive technologies program. All patients were treated for at least 2 weeks with melatonin (3 mg/day). To evaluate the cumulative effect of melatonin supplementation, we compared cycle outcomes between the first (no supplementation) and second cycles (melatonin supplementation) of patients who completed two treatment cycles. There were no significant differences in maturation rates (p = 0.50), blastocyst rates (p = 0.75), and the rate of good quality blastocysts (p = 0.59) between the first and second cycles. The fertilization rate of ICSI was higher in the second cycle than that in the first cycle (69.3 versus 77.5%). Being limited to patients with a low fertilization rate in the first cycle (<60%), the fertilization rate dramatically increased after melatonin treatment (35.1 versus 68.2%). The rate of good quality embryos also increased (48.0 versus 65.6%). An important finding in our study was that oral melatonin supplementation can have a beneficial effect on the improvement of fertilization and embryo quality and this may have occurred due to a reduction in oxidative damage.

On the basis of the good results in patients having trouble getting pregnant, one could argue that maximizing melatonin by avoiding blue light in the hours before bedtime would be beneficial to everyone, including those who wish to become pregnant.

Another 2014 paper (24996495) is titled "**Melatonin and the circadian system: contributions to**

successful female reproduction.”

The abstract reads, in part:

> Melatonin is a powerful free radical scavenger and protects the oocyte from oxidative stress, especially at the time of ovulation. The cyclic levels of melatonin in the blood pass through the placenta and aid in the organization of the fetal SCN. In the absence of this synchronizing effect, the offspring may exhibit neurobehavioral deficits. Also, melatonin protects the developing fetus from oxidative stress. Melatonin produced in the placenta likewise may preserve the optimal function of this organ.

A 2017 paper (27889913) is titled, **“Long-term melatonin treatment delays ovarian aging”**.

The abstract says in part “The present results indicate that melatonin delays ovarian aging by multiple mechanisms including antioxidant action, maintaining telomeres, stimulating SIRT expression and ribosome function, and by reducing autophagy”. Forget the details, these are all good things. The study was done in mice but the general idea applies to humans. For young women waiting to have children until a little later in life, maximizing their natural melatonin every day (night) will help preserve the quality and vitality of their eggs.

Searching pubmed.gov for "sperm melatonin" produces 189 abstracts. Almost all of them document the benefit of melatonin to the quality of sperm.

A 2014 study (25187254) is titled "**Exogenous melatonin supplementation prevents oxidative stress-evoked DNA damage in human spermatozoa.**"

> The abstract reads, in part:

> Our findings showed that the daily supplementation of 6 mg melatonin, as early as after 45 days of treatment, produced an increase in melatonin endogenous levels, indirectly measured as urinary 6-sulfatoxymelatonin (aMT6-s), an enhancement of both urinary and seminal total antioxidant capacity, and a consequent reduction in oxidative damage caused in sperm DNA. Moreover, couples whose men were given melatonin showed a statistically significant increase in the percentage of grade A, B and C at the expense of grade D embryos which were clearly reduced. In

summary, melatonin supplementation improves human sperm quality, which is essential to achieve successful natural and/or assisted reproduction outcome.

The results of a 2011 study (20964711) are stated in the title "**High endogenous melatonin concentrations enhance sperm quality and short-term in vitro exposure to melatonin improves aspects of sperm motility**." Endogenous means produced by the body.

2. Protection from brain damage

A 2014 study (24726638) of California twins is titled "**Prenatal and perinatal risk factors in a twin study of autism spectrum disorders.**" It identifies hypoxia (lack of oxygen) as the most prominent risk factor for ASD. Hypoxia can occur for many different reasons and at many different times throughout pregnancy and during birth. Melatonin has been shown in many studies to be a very effective way of protecting the brain from the damaging effect of hypoxia. We will review some of those studies

A 2016 paper (26654775) is titled "**Melatonin in Pregnancy: Effects on Brain Development and**

CNS Programming Disorders." The abstract sums up how maximizing melatonin benefits pregnancy.

Melatonin is an important neuroprotective factor and its receptors are expressed in the fetal brain. During normal pregnancy, maternal melatonin level increases progressively until term and is highly transferred to the fetus, with an important role in brain formation and differentiation. Maternal melatonin provides the first circadian signal to the fetus. This indolamine is also produced de novo and plays a protective role in the human placenta. In pregnancy disorders, both maternal and placental melatonin levels are decreased. Alteration in maternal melatonin level has been associated with disrupted brain programming with long-term effects. Melatonin has strong antioxidant protective effects directly and indirectly via the activation of its receptors. The fetal brain is highly susceptible to oxygenation variation and oxidative stress that can lead to neuronal development disruption. Based on that, several approaches have been tested as a treatment in case of pregnancy disorders and melatonin, through its neuroprotective effect, has been recently accepted against fetal brain injury. This review provides an overview about the protective effects of melatonin during pregnancy and on fetal brain development.

3. Protection from Harmful Chemicals

For a number of years there has been speculation that a chemical used in plastic called BPA may cause ASD. Since plastic is used in containers for food and water, everyone is exposed to it. A new paper (28963684) confirms that melatonin is successful in reducing potential damage to the reproductive process caused by BPA. This another reason to maximize natural melatonin.

<u>CONCLUSION</u>

Both stable circadian rhythms and cyclic melatonin availability are critical for healthy sperm and egg physiology, optimal placental function, and healthy fetal brain development. Because artificial light exposure at night disrupts the master circadian clock and suppresses nocturnal melatonin levels, light at night should be avoided. In the final chapter, we will identify simple lifestyle changes that will help parents to maximize natural melatonin production and thus minimize the risk of developing a child with Autism Spectrum Disorder.

CHAPTER 6

Lifestyle Changes to Minimize Risk for Autism

1. Regular Daily Schedule

In Chapter 2, we discussed the circadian clock and how important it is to have a robust circadian rhythm, free of disruption. While this is true for everyone, it becomes even more-so when contemplating having children. The basic idea is to make our bodies act as they did when we evolved near the equator where we experienced twelve hour of light and twelve hours of darkness every day all year round.

To develop a robust circadian rhythm one needs to maintain about the same schedule seven days a week. As the baby develops he/she will also begin developing a circadian rhythm that is synchronized with yours since the baby relies on the mother's melatonin by way of the placenta.

Getting up every morning at about the same time and exposing the eyes to light is the best way to restart the circadian clock and keep it synchronized with the rotation of the Earth. A brief exposure to daylight is probably ideal, but a brightly lit bathroom or kitchen will also work well.

Avoiding exposure of your eyes to blue light in the hours before a regular bedtime is just as important as your morning routine. Melatonin will begin flowing about 12 hours after the morning exposure to light, but only if your eyes are not exposed to blue light. Using light bulbs that don't make blue light is one way to avoid exposure. But that only works for part of the year. During the summer, it may be more practical to use glasses that block blue light to avoid evening exposure to blue light. If you wake at 7 AM, you should begin to avoid blue light at 7 PM. Use of special low blue light bulbs or orange glasses after 7 PM will maximize your natural melatonin.

2. A Good Night's Sleep

Sound sleep is important for everyone but even more-so during pregnancy. By avoiding blue light for a sufficient number of hours, melatonin production can be maximized to the 12 hours known to be possible.

A 2018 study (29101797) at Columbia University is titled, "**Blocking nocturnal blue light for insomnia: A randomized controlled trial.**" It verifies that wearing orange glasses for a few hours before bedtime improves all aspects of sleep.

Sleep experts list other things that will improve your sleep. They mention reserving your bedroom for only two things, sex and sleep. No watching TV, working on your laptop or your smart phone. Keeping your bedroom cool, dark and quiet is also conducive to sound sleep. Shades are recommended and earplugs or white noise machine to avoid distracting noise. Avoid caffeine after noon. Avoid alcohol completely even before trying to become pregnant. Stay well hydrated. Drink some water every time you use the bathroom. Frequent trips to the bathroom will not disrupt your sleep too much if you avoid exposing your eyes to blue light. Use of orange night lights will allow the flow of melatonin to continue. Avoid having your stomach either too full or too empty when you go to bed. A very light snack at bedtime may be helpful. As mentioned above, a regular schedule promotes good sleep. Toward the end of the pregnancy, sleep may be more difficult. It may be hard to find a comfortable position. Having a comfortable chair in your bedroom may offer a second place to sleep well. Asking you partner to move out for the duration is okay. Scientific studies show people sleep better by themselves. It will remove any stress you might have about your restlessness keeping him awake. If you need to turn on any lights, be sure they are low-blue or put on your blue blocking glasses.

If you have developed a strong circadian cycle your unborn baby will also experience a nighttime peak in your melatonin, which is transferred to the baby's circulation in real time. It should help your baby sleep, or be quiet while you are sleeping. Obviously this will not work 100% of the time but it should be helpful to both of you.

3. Breast-feeding

Breast-feeding is highly beneficial to both mother and child. Even if only done for a while, it provides benefits, both physical and psychological. If you are able to sustain a strong circadian cycle after the baby is born, your supply of melatonin will continue to supply your baby by way of your breast milk. As time goes on, it will help your baby develop her/his own circadian rhythm in synchrony with yours. The baby's circadian rhythm will eventually help him/her to sleep through the night!

4. Varied Diet

It is literally true …"you are what you eat". It obviously also pertains to your baby. That's why diet is so important. You need to ingest the building blocks from which your baby's body and brain will be formed. To be sure your baby gets everything he/she needs, you should greatly broaden your choice of foods. Pregnancy is not a time for picky eating or fad diets.

In addition, your doctor should prescribe a selection of vitamins and minerals. Having a consistent supply of antioxidants from fruits and vegetables protects your baby's brain from damage from lack of oxygen and other dangers. Eating lots of brightly colored fruits and vegetables throughout the day will also provide daytime melatonin and other antioxidants. Some nuts are also a good source of antioxidants.

5. Minimal Stress

If you worry too much about all of the above, that's not good for you either. Less stress also means better sleep and an easier time maintaining a daily schedule.

One needs to be realistic about having children. You do the best you can and deal with whatever happens. The power of positive thinking can't be oversold.

Conclusion.... At the end of the day

"At the end of the day" is a very popular phrase right now, so I'll use it to sum up what I hope the reader will take away from reading my book.

Autism Spectrum Disorder has become so prevalent that it touches almost everyone. It is unfortunate that we have not recognized that the use of ordinary light bulbs and all kinds of electronic devices are a probable factor in this increased incidence. It is very likely that the parents' exposure to blue light in the evening is one of the causes for this increase in ASD.

Exposure to artificial light at night from light bulbs, TV screens, computer screens, cell phones, etc. causes reduced production of natural melatonin. Melatonin is critical in producing healthy eggs and sperm. During pregnancy, if the baby's developing brain is without the protection of melatonin for even a short, but critical period of time, damage to the baby's brain may occur due to oxygen deficiency, toxins or other causes. Whether this damage can directly cause ASD is not yet understood.

The fact that there is an association between reduced melatonin and autism directly points to the benefits of maximizing melatonin. By simply avoiding blue light at night through the use of special light bulbs or blue-blocking glasses, we can

all improve our natural melatonin production. And thus, we all benefit from improved sleep, a reduction in the risk for deadly diseases, and a healthier baby with a lower risk for autism.

At the end of the day,

Without action, knowledge is of little value.